101 Tips for *Thriving* as a Chief Resident

Mel A. Ona, M.D.

Daniel R. Bashari, M.D.

Rajnish Khillan, M.D.

Foreword by:

George T. Martin, M.D., FACP
Chairman, Department of Medicine
Lutheran Medical Center
Brooklyn, N.Y.

101 Tips for *Thriving* as a Chief Resident

101 Tips for *Thriving* as a Chief Resident
ISBN-13: 978-1475228274
ISBN-10: 1475228279

Printed in the United States of America.

The authors would like to thank:

Our families for their unconditional love and support.

Dr. George T. Martin *for giving us the opportunity to thrive as Chief Residents.*

Dr. Daniel Giaccio *for lending insights and invaluable tips that made our job more enjoyable and fulfilling.*

Dr. Ravi Gupta *for teaching us how to become better teachers ourselves.*

Ms. Eileen Kruck *for your expertise and daily support.*

Foreword

Your Chief Residency will be a year of enormous professional and personal growth, a time when you not only broaden your own medical knowledge and teaching skills, but more importantly, when you hone your interpersonal skills. It is the year when you learn the important lessons necessary to succeed in your career. The ability to deal effectively with a wide variety of challenges and personalities may well be the most demanding, and satisfying, skill to master. Your Chief Residency is a year of supporting and reassuring, of negotiating and mediating, a year of mentoring and being mentored, of teaching and being taught, of growing and helping others grow. In short, it will be the best year of your residency.

At the same time it may be the most difficult and frightening year of your life. It is like parenting; there are no easy answers to the myriad problems you will be forced to confront. Your Chair and Program Director are relying on you, yet the Chief Residency may be the job you feel least prepared for.

That is why I wish I had this book when I was a Chief Resident. It is full of invaluable advice and is a guide you will refer to frequently throughout the year. It describes the strategies and interpersonal skills you need to succeed as a Chief Resident and steers you away from the pitfalls that many find themselves falling into. Because they have mastered these techniques, the authors are destined for success, and if you heed their suggestions, and warnings, you will be also.

George T. Martin, M.D., FACP
Chairman, Department of Medicine
Lutheran Medical Center
Brooklyn, N.Y.

Chief Resident, 1974 - 1975
Bellevue Hospital
New York, N.Y.

Note: We were Chief Residents during our PGY-3 year, but these tips are just as practical and valuable for PGY-4 (or higher) Chief Residents

---

1.) You will not please everyone all the time.

Understand this from day one. Some residents will love you and others will denounce you. Whenever you work with a group of people, know that many of them may not realize that you are considering many different inputs. At times, difficult decisions must be made that will not be agreeable to everyone. As long as your residents see and understand that you have considered their ideas, communicated and worked with them towards the best decision (or even the least worst alternative!) they will respect you.

2.) Always protect your residents.

You are the residents' advocate. They expect you to fight for them and they deserve it.

3.) Be seen.

Walk around throughout the units and wards so that residents get a chance to speak to you one-on-one. You will be viewed as more approachable and proactive.

4.) Conduct resident-only meetings

This gives residents a chance to be open and honest with any and all issues. Some residency programs hold house staff meetings primarily with the Program Director or Department Chair, however, having resident-only meetings may encourage more open discussion.

5.) Always propose ways to improve the program.

Your Program Director, Department Chair, and residents will see that you care about the program and the program will improve overall.

6.) Find the fairest and quickest way to resolve issues between residents.

Working through issues promptly and fairly will boost morale and assuage ongoing conflicts.

7.) Promote camaraderie in the program.

Schedule fun, social activities, such as dinners, games, and general get-togethers. This enables the residents to get to know each other outside of work, find common interests, create deeper bonds of friendship, and ultimately will help with building a better team environment.

8.) Be a model resident.

The residents look up to you. Strive to be the best – this will inspire other residents to excel.

9.) Address issues as they arise.

Addressing issues as they arise as opposed to letting them pile up will ensure that you won't miss important things. Your job is multi-faceted. Be decisive and disciplined with daily tasks/problems. Otherwise, you'll end up floundering and falling far behind.

10.) Create the resident schedule according to ACGME guidelines.

Always review the most updated ACGME policies as they apply to resident scheduling. The schedule/curriculum may change and you must be vigilant with maintaining compliance with the ACGME mandates.

11.) Have a list of resident's contact information available at all times.

When residents are absent due to illness or an emergency, your contact list will be vital for obtaining coverage.

12.) Be available.

Be available via cell phone, email, pager, and of course, in person. Residents, Attendings, hospital staff, and the

Administration rely on you to be available at all times for assistance and troubleshooting.

13.) Dress well.

Impressions count. Being well dressed at all times solidifies the perception of maturity and professionalism that others will have of you.

14.) Be professional always and in all ways.

In person, on the phone, via email, in writing, through actions—you never know who's watching or noticing.

15.) Obtain feedback from your peers regarding what you could be doing better.

You may be blinded to your own limitations. Seeking feedback keeps you sharp and shows commitment to constant and never-ending improvement.

16.) Be authentic and be yourself.
Your uniqueness enriches the program.

17.) Attend national conferences or faculty development sessions.
These meetings/sessions enhance knowledge, leadership skills, and interpersonal growth.

18.) Incorporate active participation from residents and medical students in morning report.
Morning report should be about delving into a case and critically thinking through it, all the way through from presentation to diagnosis and treatment. The more active the

participation, the better will be the learning process and everyone will remember the case more clearly. More importantly, the residents will then use the information to improve their clinical management skills.

19.) Plan and lead separate teaching sessions with medical students.

Schedule at least one hour per day to meet with a group of medical students and go over topics. You'll retain more knowledge when you teach.

20.) Keep an open door policy for the residents.

Residents will seek your counsel about work, personal matters, and life in general. You will often be called upon to be an emotional support and anchor for troubled house staff.

21.) Reprimand problem residents privately and discretely.

Doing so will maintain peace.

22.) Be present at all resident meetings.

Graduate Medical Education meetings, House Staff Association meetings, Fact Findings, Morbidity/Mortality meetings, and other Committee meetings etc. will benefit from your participation and leadership.

23.) Work closely with the program coordinator.

He/she is a tremendous resource and support system throughout the year.

24.) Check in regularly with the Program Director and Department Chair.

You are a direct link and voice of the residents.

25.) Be first to attend all conferences, lectures, Grand Rounds, etc.

You must set the example and not only be on time for all conferences/lectures but also you are responsible for keeping attendance.

26.) Keep your cool in the face of conflict and crisis.

While there will be times when residents/attendings may "get under your skin" or perhaps treat you with great disrespect, you must remain composed. Step away if you must, but always stay calm, cool, and collected. This skill is very challenging and difficult to do but it will save you TONS of heartache by preventing you from saying or doing something you might regret later.

27.) Always hear both sides of the story.

People will appreciate your impartiality and fairness in the midst of conflict. Don't rush to judgment without listening to all the facts from all sides first.

28.) Commit to expanding your knowledge base by reading (i.e. journal articles, books, etc.) on a daily basis.

Reading sharpens your intellect and makes you more well-rounded.

29.) Leave bad feelings at work (and let them go!).

Life is too short to harbor negativity. Let it go or at the very least, leave it at work.

30.) Escalate problems to the Program Director and/or Chair if you cannot resolve the issue.

Some residents will be extremely stubborn and will not listen nor heed your authority. At this point, escalate the problem right away to establish professional boundaries. Otherwise, your residents will continue to be subordinate.

31.) Learn how to communicate with different social styles and respect all cultures.

Residents will come from all points of the globe. Learning how to be a "social chameleon" will serve you well, not only with building rapport with others, but also when dealing with conflict.

32.) Encourage creativity and promote solutions for making the residency program better.

Tell your residents that complaints will be heard...but solutions to those complaints will make things better. Encourage them to come up with their own solutions for particular problems.

33.) Meet with other Chief Residents from other services (Surgery, Family Medicine, Ob/Gyn, etc.) to learn how they have worked through challenges in their own programs.

You can help each other avoid mistakes made in certain situations and come up with novel solutions by thinking "outside the box."

34.) Enjoy the work.

Not everyone has the ability or opportunity to be a Chief Resident. Many programs hold this position with great distinction. Be proud of the accomplishment and stay focused on the goal of improving every day.

35.) Give others credit for solving problems.

This builds rapport and morale for the program. It also enhances confidence in that resident.

36.) Teach more often.

Seek out opportunities to teach residents and medical students. Lead teaching rounds in the morning. Conduct morning report whenever possible. This will hone your knowledge base and improve your communication/teaching skills.

37.) Attend the ACGME Chief Resident conference.

You will meet other rising Chief Residents from programs around the nation in all different specialties (e.g. Anesthesia, OB/Gyn, Surgery, Radiology, Pathology, etc.) and learn in an interactive way how to become a more effective leader. Plus, you'll meet and network with many other like-minded, excellence-pursuing, residents such as yourself.

38.) Subscribe to the American College of Physician's Chief Resident's corner online.

You'll benefit from myriad resources to help you in your day-to-day duties.

39.) Keep track of as many details as possible regarding resident calls, schedules, shifts, holidays worked, etc.

Residents will be keeping meticulous track of when they've worked, whom they've worked with, and how often they've been on call. The more you accurately keep track of things the fairer will be the process of delegating calls (especially the least desirable ones!).

40.) Fill in when necessary for emergency calls.

Emergencies happen. Be the one to step up when no one else can or is willing.

41.) Find an outlet for daily stressors.

*Exercise regularly, get enough sleep, eat well, foster your talents, spend time with family. These outlets will keep you sane when things get rough (and they **will** get rough!).*

42.) Be fair but stand firm when residents resist necessary change.

Be an advocate and support the residents, however, you are also a liaison for the department and for administration. Communicate with residents up front and promptly regarding policy changes as soon as they are implemented.

43.) **Communicate with your residents daily.**

Keep them informed and stay in touch via email and in person. They will see that you are a resource to help and support them.

44.) **Be proactive.**

Ask residents, "How's everything going?" And "What can I do to help you today?"

45.) **Hone your clinical skills.**

Being a Chief Resident is not always about being an administrator. Choose rotations/electives that will prepare and enable you to care for patients. You are a doctor first.

46.) Work with nursing to enhance communication among physicians and the nursing staff.

Nurses are the lifeblood of any hospital. Keep things smooth between residents and nursing staff—you'll find that the quality of patient care will thrive.

47.) Don't take it personally when residents claim that "our Chiefs have NO power!"

Fact #1: Chief Residents have <u>considerable</u> influence. The best Chiefs keep a delicate balance with managing their own training, helping to run the training program, and maintaining the best interests *of the residents. Keeping track of everyone's personal and professional requests is a daunting task—even more difficult is trying to execute of all of these requests.*

Fact #2: Perception is reality. Whether or not your peers think you have "power" is irrelevant. Your goal is not to change their minds nor prove anyone wrong. Stick to the common goal of constant and never-ending improvement for yourself, your program, and the relationships among all professionals, students, and staff in the institution.

48.) Keep in touch with all the other Chiefs.

Let the other Chiefs know whenever requests are made and changes are implemented. Open communication is best.

49.) Don't undermine the other Chiefs.

Again, keep communication lines open. If one Chief makes a change without telling the other Chief(s), this can easily lead to conflict. Residents can manipulate the situation and continue to "go to the nice Chief" rather than deal with the "strict Chief"—this can complicate matters significantly.

50.) Have a weekly meeting with the other Chief Residents.

Discussing all issues will keep transitions smooth.

51.) Maximize the other Chief Residents' talents.

One Chief may be a genius with scheduling. The other may be a master communicator who can defuse resident conflicts instantly. Another may have a superior organizational mind and contribute by creating systems for keeping track of everything—whatever the case, work synergistically and collaboratively.

52.) Be honest—always and in all ways!

Your integrity and honesty are reflections of your character. Be honest. Don't ruin your integrity and character by lying or covering up issues.

53.) Maintain professionalism among your colleagues (if you are a PGY-3 Chief Resident).

Some residents will not accept the fact that you are a selected leader among the group. Remain humble and professional and reduce your association with negative and insubordinate colleagues. Escalate problems when necessary.

54.) Work with problem residents.

You may be appointed to tutor/monitor/work with struggling residents. Do your best to guide them and keep administration informed regarding their progress.

55.) Find a mentor and keep in touch with him/her on a consistent basis.

Having a coach will keep you focused and on your game. Your mentor will inspire you towards excellence.

56.) Keep in touch with past Chiefs.

They can be your greatest asset and resource. They've already "been there, done that" and they can help you learn from their mistakes. They are always willing to help (that's why they were Chiefs before!).

57.) Be humble.

Don't let the title get to your head. It's a privileged position and can be abused. Having humility and staying grounded will ensure that you lead with fairness and compassion.

58.) Be wary of resident cliques.

It's human nature for people to group together. Be wary of those resident groups who simply gossip and grumble. Don't waste your time and energy with what they say.

Treat them as fairly as you would all other residents but don't let the clique overrun the program. Communicate up-front with the administration and with all the other residents. This will keep the cliques in check. Your job is to represent ALL residents regarding the program. Words and gossip don't count. Actions and implementation of policy do.

59.) Remember, when dealing with the worst crises...this, too, shall pass.

Maintain perspective. Your time as Chief Resident is finite. You have the rest of your medical career ahead. Even in the face of failure and heartache, you will get through!

60.) Provide feedback on your junior residents' and medical students' performance.

They will appreciate it and they will get a good sense of where they stand.

61.) Follow all hospital "red rules" and enforce them when these red rules are broken. (E.g. patient identification, time out protocol, central line bundle, etc.)

You are an administrative agent who is obligated to follow and enforce the "red rules" of your institution. These "red rules" preserve patient safety—and you must make patient safety a top priority.

62.) Be respectful of all patients and their family members in the hospital.

You are a representative of your hospital and patients want to feel comfortable being here or having their family member here.

63.) Realize that you are a liaison to the attendings and other staff.

You have a unique position as a liaison and mediator. You have residents who will look up to you and you have the administration that expects you to convey and communicate policies to the house staff.

64.) Have all contact information for residents, attendings, administrators, and hospital personnel on hand—especially the numbers for on-call personnel.

You will get frequent pages and calls from operators and other staff who need to know who is on-call or available. You are the point person. Be prepared with all pertinent contact information—it'll make your life much easier.

65.) Check all conference presentations ahead of time, and ensure that Audiovisual support is on site and be ready for any problems that may arise.

There's nothing more embarrassing than having an auditorium full of people watching you trying (and failing) to load an important presentation for a prestigious speaker. (Don't let this happen.)

66.) Be respectful of all attending physicians' contact information.

Check and double check which phone numbers attendings would like to have listed.

67.) Honor confidential information.

As a Chief Resident, you will be entrusted with sensitive and often privileged information – keep it confidential!

68.) Propose innovative ideas and commit to systems improvements.

You are an integral part of the residency program as a resident leader and advocate. Your ideas may tangibly improve the program now and in the future.

69.) Keep up to date with ACGME requirements.

This will serve you and the program well when milestones documentation is required and when site visits occur.

70.) **Don't be a know-it-all**

No one likes a know-it-all. (See Tip #57)

71.) **Respond to all codes within the hospital.**

Be there to assist with any problems. In fact, you may be the first responder to the code/emergency. Realize that everyone is there to help and if you can coordinate all available personnel, this can lead to positive outcomes.

72.) **Keep a journal of your challenges and experiences.**

Your year will be filled with myriad experiences, some small and seemingly insignificant, and others may be life altering. It's true that if life is worth living, then it's worth recording.

73.) Call back right away when you are paged.

This reflects your commitment to professionalism.

74.) Develop thick skin, but be a sensitive listener at the same time.

Stay steadfast, fair, and professional. Having this quality will prepare you well for professional life after residency.

75.) Don't procrastinate.

The urge to procrastinate is directly proportional to the amount of stress you will encounter. You have the power to manipulate this equation— less procrastination equals less stress. Get things done now that you can put off tomorrow!

76.) Tell yourself this affirmation aloud every day, *"I GET to do this and live my dream of being the best Chief Resident I can be". (You'll actually feel a positive difference. Trust us...try it!)*

77.) Prepare all resident schedules in a timely fashion.
> *Doing so will prevent residents from constantly approaching you to find out what their next rotation is. Also, the residents need their schedules ahead of time so that they can make personal future plans (e.g. travel, interviews, etc.)*

78.) Keep a sense of humor.
> *It will help you maintain perspective and stay buoyant when crises arise or when difficult or vindictive people try to pull you down.*

79.) Be prepared to break bad news.

Occasionally, you may be called upon to discipline a resident or give bad news to personnel. Breaking bad news in a professional and composed manner will prepare you in the future. (It will never be easy but you can learn how to be more compassionate and composed.)

80.) Understand your multi-faceted role.

You are a leader, coach, moderator, teacher, motivator, listener, friend, mentor, physician, administrator, liaison, and confidant.

81.) You are Chief Resident for the ENTIRE academic year.

Despite the fact that you may not have active Chief

responsibilities for a particular month, be willing to help even if you're not officially assigned – residents will know that you always care about their interests.

82.) Have each other's backs!
Cooperation, communication, and seamless cross coverage among your co-Chiefs will ensure organization and smooth operations for each other and the program.

83.) Conduct weekly board review sessions with other residents.
This activity will help you and your residents gain more confidence and fortify an essential knowledge foundation before sitting for the boards.

84.) Volunteer for service-oriented, extra-curricular activities.

Spending quality time as a volunteer enhances your interpersonal skills and helps you develop into a well-rounded and altruistic physician.

85.) Always address / report lapses in patient care.

For example, if a code (e.g. Rapid Response Team or cardiac arrest code) is called and the necessary participating staff show up late (or don't show up at all) you must address this promptly and firmly, so that it doesn't occur again. Patient safety and care are at stake and are apriori!

86.) Choose a variety of topics for afternoon lectures and organize them in a logical way.

Schedule lectures early in the academic year that address diagnostic and treatment approaches to common hospital conditions. This will enable the new house staff to apply what they have learned in these practical lectures to the patients they are caring for.

87.) When teaching, encourage active participation among residents and medical students in a constructive, non-threatening way.

Learning becomes understanding when active participation is encouraged in a non-malignant manner (i.e. no "pimping"). The goal must be on the process of critical thinking rather than getting the "right answer." Lead the

*residents and students through
the thinking process so that the
goal is learning and not "being
right" all the time.*

88.) Listen to every complaint without interruption.

*Residents will complain about
almost everything. They will
appreciate your ability to listen
without judgment. Resist the
urge to cut the resident off
when they bring up the same
complaint over and over again.
Understand that some
residents complain because it
helps them feel better.*

89.) Inquire and provide interesting cases that may be presented at a Morbidity and Mortality conference.

*We all learn valuable lessons
from patient cases that are not*

managed well. Also, these cases may serve as opportunities to create systems improvements and improve patient safety in the future.

90.) Always share rare and interesting cases with other residents and attendings in the hospital.

Remember your role as teacher. Rare and interesting cases deepen one's clinical perspective and stimulate discussion and collaboration among other services and disciplines.

91.) When choosing cases for morning report, complexity should increase over the academic year.

Early on, choose a variety of commonly seen conditions (e.g. heart failure, acute myocardial infarction, syncope, pneumonia, asthma/COPD, diarrhea, etc.) so that new residents will feel confident in managing patients who present with these illnesses. As the weeks and months pass, choose more complex cases to build upon what the residents have already learned and applied.

92.) Organize alumni events to keep in touch with graduates from your program.

This creates excellent networking opportunities and strengthens the support system for graduates-to-be who are seeking new employment or career advice from those already established.

93.) Create and run a Medical "Jeopardy!"*-style game periodically throughout the year.

This is incredibly fun and encourages active learning through entertainment and friendly competition.

94.) Reinforce the importance of required documentation in admission notes, progress notes, consultations, and discharge summary dictations among the residents.

This is a very important point that is often overlooked. Good documentation (e.g. date/time of every note, procedure notes, thorough assessment/plans, etc.) improves patient care and decreases risk of litigation.

95.) Emphasize the importance of managing length of stay.

Preventing extra days that patients spend in the hospital will reduce their risk for nosocomial infection and prevent unnecessary medical costs. Managing length of stay is directly related to ensuring that work is done efficiently and collaboratively (i.e. physicians, nurses, case managers, social workers, consultants, physical therapists, etc.).

96.) Support your co-Chiefs when disciplinary action is administered to residents.

This is especially important if the disciplined resident is a friend of one of the Chief Residents. (Remember Tip #49)

97.) Propose research ideas for residents and medical students.

Many residents and students may not know where to start in terms of research opportunities or how to get involved with existing projects. You can encourage the residents and students to assist with your own project(s) or help them formulate a proposal to begin their own research study.

98.) Give positive feedback (both in person and in public) and excellent evaluations for residents that do a great job.

Reinforcing good behavior helps to perpetuate it. Giving positive feedback publicly also enhances morale among the residents. It also makes the stronger residents continue to serve as excellent examples for others to emulate and model.

47

99.) Don't do everything yourself.
Master the ability of delegation—to leverage the efforts of others. You'll get much more work done this way and save time as well.

100.) Keep your beeper on 24/7.
You are a point person with influence, connections, and considerable responsibility. Be reliable and available because you may be called upon in an emergency.

101.) Train and support the new, rising Chief Residents!
Towards the end of the academic year, meet with the new, rising chiefs and give them a complete rundown of everything they will be managing. (And don't forget to provide them a copy of this book! ☺)

ABOUT THE AUTHORS

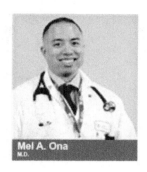

Mel A. Ona, M.D., M.S., M.P.H., M.A.

Dr. Ona was born in Boston, MA and raised in Rochester, NY. Prior to medical school he attended graduate school in Boston and received three Masters Degrees. He has published three books, founded several websites such as www.MelOna.com, and www.OnaHealthyLife.com, recorded two music CDs, and earned two black belts (JKD/Doce Pares), and a blue belt (Brazilian Jiu Jitsu). He graduated from St. George's University School of Medicine and was the recipient of the White Coat Award. After Chief Residency, Dr. Ona will be working as a hospitalist and then entering a fellowship in Gastroenterology.

ABOUT THE AUTHORS

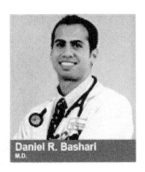

Daniel R. Bashari
M.D.

Daniel R. Bashari, M.D.

Dr. Bashari was born and raised on Long Island, New York. He attended Ross University School of Medicine where he graduated with High Honors. As a second year resident at Lutheran, Dan participated in an original research project in the treatment of patients with congestive heart failure that resulted in a reduction in the incidence of re-admissions to the hospital. This research became the Best Research Project of the Year for 2011 in Internal Medicine at Lutheran Medical Center and was subsequently published in a peer-reviewed medical journal. After graduation, he will be entering a Geriatric Fellowship and then pursuing a career in Hospitalist Medicine.

ABOUT THE AUTHORS

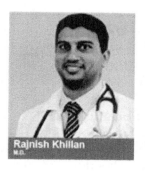

Rajnish Khillan, M.D.

Dr. Khillan was born and raised in Punjab, India. He attended the Government Medical College at Nagpur where he graduated with Highest Honors. As a PGY-2, he presented posters for his research at several national conferences including the American College of Physicians, American Medical Association, American Heart Association, American Society of Clinical Oncology, and the Medical Society for the State of New York. After graduation, Rajnish will be pursuing a career in Hospitalist Medicine.

Tip Index

* "Jeopardy!" is a registered trademark of Jeopardy Productions, Inc.

Notes

_____

_____

_____

_____

_____

_____

_____

_____

_____

_____

_____

_____

_____

_____

_____

_____

Notes

_____

_____

_____

_____

_____

_____

_____

_____

_____

_____

_____

_____

_____

_____

Notes

Notes

_____

_____

_____

_____

_____

_____

_____

_____

_____

_____

_____

_____

_____

_____

_____

_____

Notes

_____

_____

_____

_____

_____

_____

_____

_____

_____

_____

_____

_____

_____

_____

_____

_____

Notes

_____

_____

_____

_____

_____

_____

_____

_____

_____

_____

_____

_____

_____

_____

_____

_____

_____

_____

Notes

Notes

_____

_____

_____

_____

_____

_____

_____

_____

_____

_____

_____

_____

_____

_____

_____

_____

Notes

_____

_____

_____

_____

_____

_____

_____

_____

_____

_____

_____

_____

_____

_____

_____

_____

Made in the USA
Coppell, TX
30 April 2020